Chair Yoga for You
A Practical Guide

Clarissa C. Adkins, Olivette Baugh Robinson & Barbara Leaf Stewart

Photography by Mary Davis

www.chairyogaforyou.com

Copyright © 2011 Clarissa C. Adkins, Olivette Baugh Robinson, Barbara Leaf Stewart
All rights reserved.

ISBN: 1456324500
ISBN-13: 9781456324506
Library of Congress Control Number: 2010916650

ABOUT THE AUTHORS AND CONTRIBUTERS

Clarissa C. Adkins

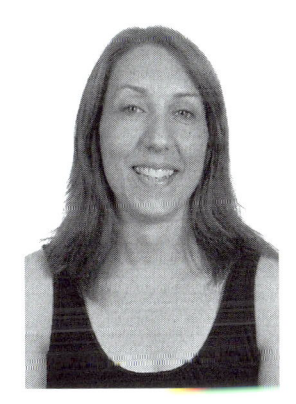

Clarissa is YogaFit trained, RYT 200 (Registered Yoga Teacher), with a passion for the study of all styles of yoga, especially Ashtanga and Iyengar. Her background includes a BA in English from James Madison University (1997), teaching English in Japan, and learning yoga from her father starting at age 14. She spends time coordinating yoga classes, teaching yoga, and freelance writing. Much of her writing appears on Livestrong.com. In 2010, she celebrated her five-year anniversary as a yoga instructor. Clarissa thanks those who have inspired her on her yoga path, including Jasper C. and Verena V. Lupo, Lawrence Lupo, Jeanne Wheeler, Arlene Bjork and Olivette Robinson.

Olivette Baugh Robinson

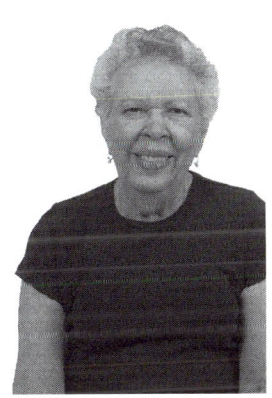

Olivette was born in Petersburg, Virginia, in 1925. She received a MA degree in Early Childhood Education from NYU in 1953. After enjoying a long career as the director of a day care center in Brooklyn, New York, Olivette discovered yoga. In 1994, she took the month-long teacher training course to become a certified Sivananda Yoga instructor. She began teaching yoga classes and chair yoga classes in senior centers in Queens, New York. Having moved to Midlothian, Virginia, she introduced chair yoga to one of the YMCAs in 2001. Olivette continues teaching yoga, chair yoga, gentle yoga, and kids yoga at YMCAs, a retirement community, and a senior center. At age 86, she feels blessed to be able to continue teaching yoga. Olivette wishes to thank Theresa Price for teaching her yoga and chair yoga.

Barbara Leaf Stewart

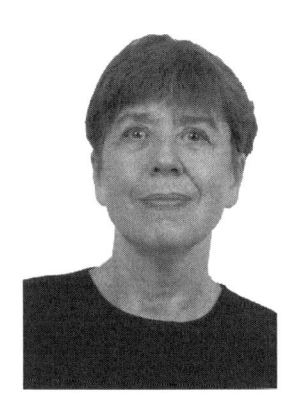

Barbara has an MS in Physiology from Florida State University. During her thirty-year career in college teaching at J. Sargeant Reynolds Community College (Professor Emeritus), she worked on the national, regional, and local level advancing science education and teacher preparation. Her yoga practice began in 1985. Retirement gave her the opportunity to fulfill her long-term dream and complete the Teacher Training Course at the International Sivananda Yoga Vedanta Centre (RYT 200). Barbara currently teaches yoga in the Richmond, Virginia, region. She thanks her mentor Olivette Robinson, her yoga community, and her students for helping her continually deepen her yoga practice.

Herb Baugh, Model

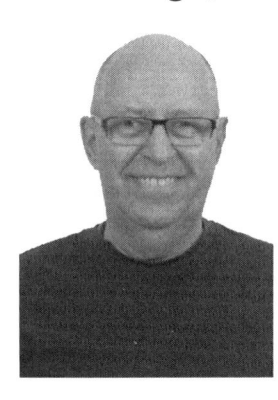

Herb enjoyed his years as a pilot and flight instructor. At age 54, Herb became aware of the many benefits of yoga while taking yoga classes on Long Island, New York. He is pleased that he introduced his sister Olivette to yoga.

Mary Davis, Photographer

Mary's passion is photography. After nearly ten years of photography and art experience, she began her own business as a professional photographer. She specializes in wedding and portrait photography in the Richmond, Virginia, and surrounding areas.

ACKNOWLEDGMENTS

We are grateful for the advice, contributions, patience, and knowledge we received from family, friends, teachers and colleagues, especially the following individuals: Linda McDorman, for helping us get this project started; Mark, Katherine, Daniel, and Eric Adkins, for their continued love, patience, and support; Eric Davis, for helping us with babysitting during photo sessions; Eric, Nita, and Ashley Baugh, for their review of medical-related content; David P. Baugh, for legal advice; Kevin Stewart, for recommending CreateSpace; Demand Studios, for the generous grant and encouragement; and to our yoga students, for providing us with the inspiration to take on and complete this endeavor.

CONTENTS

	Page
WELCOME	13
HOW TO USE THIS BOOK	14
PRINCIPLES OF YOGA	14
PRECAUTIONS	15
BREATHING EXERCISES	17
ABDOMINAL BREATHING	17
COMPLETE BREATH	18
ALTERNATE NOSTRIL BREATHING I	18
ALTERNATE NOSTRIL BREATHING II	18
ALTERNATE NOSTRIL BREATHING III	19
HOW TO BEGIN	20
SITTING POSTURES	20
DRISHTI	21
BREATHING AND RELAXING	21
INTENTION	21
WARM-UP POSTURES	23
TORSO	23
1. CAT/COW	23
2. FLOWING AIRPLANE	24
3. FLOWING SPINAL TWIST	24
4. CIRCLING ARMS	25

UPPER BODY 26
   5. SHOULDER SHRUGS 26
   6. SHOULDER ROLLS 26
   7. SHOULDER RELEASE 26
   8. SIDE-TO-SIDE NECK WARM-UP 27
   9. TURTLE NECK 27
  10. NECK PENDULUM 27
  11. HALF MOON 28

LOWER BODY 29
  12. KNEE LIFTS 29
  13. KNEE CROSS AND ROTATE 30
  14. KNEE TO CHEST 31
  15. LEG EXTENSIONS 31
  16. ANKLE ROTATIONS 32
  17. TOE AND HEEL TAPPING 32
  18. FOOT ROTATIONS 33
  19. FOOT PRESSES 33
  20. SUN SALUTATION 33

ENDURANCE AND
STRENGTH POSTURES **34**
  SEATED POSTURES 34
  21. CHAIR POSE 34
  22. ARM CIRCLES 35
  23. TRIANGLE 35
  24. PRAYER SQUAT FLOW 36
  25. ELBOW TO KNEE 37
  26. REVOLVED TRIANGLE 37
  27. WARRIOR I 38
  28. WARRIOR II 38
  29. REVERSED WARRIOR 39
  30. SIDE-ANGLE WARRIOR 39
  31. CAMEL 40

32.	GATE	40
33.	EAGLE	41
34.	CHEST EXPANSION	42
35.	SPINAL TWIST	42

STANDING POSTURES — 43

36.	MOUNTAIN POSE	43
37.	CAT/COW	44
38.	ARM CIRCLES	45
39.	PRAYER SQUAT FLOW	46
40.	HALF MOON	47
41.	TRIANGLE	48
42.	REVOLVED TRIANGLE	49
43.	WARRIOR I	49
44.	WARRIOR II	50
45.	REVERSED WARRIOR	50
46.	SIDE-ANGLE WARRIOR	51
47.	CAMEL	51
48.	DOWNDOG	52
49.	LEG RAISE	52
50.	FORWARD BEND	53

BALANCE POSTURES — 54

51.	BALANCE ON TOES	55
52.	FLAMINGO	55
53.	KNEE LIFTS	55
54.	KNEE TO CHEST	56
55.	KNEE UP TWIST	56
56.	TREE	57
57.	DANCER'S POSE	58
58.	DANCER WITH HALF BOW	58
59.	WARRIOR III	59
60.	CHAIR SQUAT	59
61.	CHAIR SQUAT ON ONE LEG	60

COOL-DOWN POSTURES 61
62. BACK OF SHOULDER STRETCH 61
63. MIDDLE OF BACK STETCH 62
64. ROCK THE BABY 62
65. PIGEON 63
66. HAMSTRING STRETCH 63
67. INNER THIGH STRETCH 64
68. WRIST RELEASE 64
69. FACIAL RELEASE 64
70. LION POSE 65
71. SEATED FORWARD BEND 65

FINGER EXERCISES 66
72. FINGER FLEX 66
73. FINGER SQUEEZE 66
74. FINGER STRETCHES 66
75. PULL AND TWIST 66
76. JOINING 66
77. PARTING 66
78. THUMB TO FINGERS 66

FOOT AND TOE EXERCISES 67
79. PULL AND TWIST 67
80. MASSAGE 67
81. CLASP 67

EYE EXERCISES 68
82. UP-DOWN RIGHT-LEFT 68
83. DIAGONAL RIGHT-LEFT 68
84. AROUND THE CLOCK 68
85. FINGER GAZE 68
86. COVERED EYES 68

FINAL RELAXATION AND MEDITATION **69**
   PREPARING TO RELAX 69
   RELAXING BODY AND MIND 69
   MEDITATION 70
   NAMASTE 72

APPENDIX **73**

SAMPLE SESSIONS **73**

SANSKRIT NAMES **79**

RESOURCES **81**

WELCOME

> *You are younger today than you will ever be again.*
> *Make the most of it for tomorrow.*
> —Anon

Chair yoga is part of the hatha branch of yoga. Hatha relates to yoga of the body, including poses, breathing, and meditation. Yoga techniques help you create a better harmony between your body, mind, and spirit. They also provide you with a low-impact way to increase strength, flexibility, and balance, while teaching you how relax.

In chair yoga students practice poses while seated in a chair or use the chair for assistance in some standing poses. Anyone can practice it. Those with chronic conditions, weight issues, past injuries, disabilities, or anyone looking for gradual and gentle ways to increase his or her range of motion can all experience benefits from this practice. Chair yoga is also appropriate for students of more traditional yoga classes who want to rediscover poses that they long ago committed to muscle memory. In other words, people of all ages, levels, and physical conditions are able to start a chair yoga practice without hesitation.

In creating this book, we sought to incorporate the needs of students studying on their own, as well as those wishing to design their own chair yoga classes. We are hopeful these pages will express our belief that anyone and everyone can discover the beauty and benefits of yoga, whether using chair yoga as a starting place or as an addition to their mind and body fitness routine. Additionally, we encourage you

WELCOME

to seek out yoga classes in your area so you can enjoy the group setting. It is our goal that all yoga students discover one of the simplest rewards of yoga: being able to function through life's daily activities and demands with ease of movement and peace of mind.

HOW TO USE THIS BOOK

We encourage you to read through the following paragraphs, which outline the principles of yoga, precautions, and how to begin your practice.

Additionally, take a little time to read over the breathing exercises and poses before practicing them so your experience is more fluid. Accompanying most poses are photos to help you visualize the written descriptions. We divided the yoga exercises into the following categories:

- Breathing Exercises
- Warm-up Postures
- Endurance and Strength Postures
- Balance Postures
- Cool-down Postures

At the end of this book, we include several sequences, or combinations of poses, for a practice of at least thirty minutes. You can also design your own sequences as you become more comfortable with the poses. Always start with a few poses from the warm-up section and end with a few from the cool-down postures. Because the universal language of yoga is Sanskrit, you will also find an index at the end of this book with English to Sanskrit translations of poses.

PRINCIPLES of YOGA

Although the following five principles encompass ideas from all styles of yoga, they originate from Sivananda, as taught by Swami Vishnu-devananda in *The Complete Illustrated Book of Yoga*:

WELCOME

1. PROPER EXERCISE: Yoga exercises are performed slowly, gently, and with awareness. Keep in mind that all bodies are different.

2. PROPER BREATHING: Deep breathing helps to nourish and strengthen the body.

3. PROPER RELAXATION: Releasing tension through relaxation is essential for a healthy body. Many yoga students consider complete relaxation of the body and mind to be most difficult, but important to work toward.

4. PROPER DIET: Simple, nutritious foods are basic for good health. A true yoga diet is a vegetarian diet.

5. POSITIVE THINKING and MEDITATION: Positive thinking leads to contentment — being thankful for who you are, what you can do, and what you have. There is no need to envy what others can do or what others have. Make peace with the past and move forward.

> *The body is as young as the spine is flexible.*
> —Old yogic saying

PRECAUTIONS

As much as chair yoga is a gentle, safe road to take toward fitness, *please follow the advice of your physician on exercises that you should or should not do.*

Yoga emphasizes "listening to the body." The exercises and poses are sometimes challenging, but should never be practiced to the point of pain. There are many ways to achieve the same stretch or the same objective in yoga, so always feel free to skip a pose and move on to the next one. Before doing any endurance exercises or deep stretches, please warm up.

Pay special attention to the following conditions:

Disc issues or spinal degeneration – When bending forward from the waist, go only about 45 degrees (not chest to thighs).

Spinal arthritis/bone spurs and degeneration – When bending backward, keep the head straight rather than allowing the head to fall back.

High or low blood pressure – On postures that move the head and/or chest up or down, move slowly to allow for the body to adjust to the change.

The above is a list of the most common contraindications. Most importantly, listen to your body and your physician.

BREATHING EXERCISES

> *Breath is life.*
> —Krishnamacharya

Correct breathing is one of yoga's key principles. The outcome of relaxation can quickly be obtained through basic breathing exercises. It also helps you maintain focus, heat in the body, and good circulation throughout your practice. These exercises are also beneficial for the respiratory, circulatory, and nervous systems.

Yoga breathing is usually done through the nostrils, which helps keep heat in the body as opposed to most aerobic exercise where you usually exhale through the mouth to help cool the body.

Keep in mind that when one is becoming accustomed to breathing techniques, it is common to become a bit light-headed, dizzy, or tense. Try these techniques a little at a time and with a relaxed and open mind. If you experience anything uncomfortable, then stop and try again another time.

ABDOMINAL BREATHING

Inhale deeply through your nose. Allow the abdomen to expand, which helps lower your diaphragm, and bring oxygen into the base of the lungs. Exhale through your nose. Contract your abdominal muscles, pull your abdomen in, and raise the diaphragm, pushing out air.

If this is new to you it will feel awkward at first. Try the exercise while lying on your back with one hand over your belly button. Feel the rise and fall of your abdomen.

COMPLETE BREATH

Beginning with the abdominal breath, focus on this outward and inward movement of the belly for a few breaths. When this feels comfortable, focus on bringing this expansion upward toward the chest on the inhale as if you were filling up a pitcher with water. On the exhalations, the water is draining out of the pitcher.

ALTERNATE NOSTRIL BREATHING I

You can experiment with many variations of Alternate Nostril Breathing. Here is one of the simpler versions: Hold up your right hand. Fold down your index and middle fingers. You will use your thumb and fingers to gently seal your nostrils closed. Close off your right nostril with your thumb while you inhale through your left nostril. Close off your left nostril with your fingers. Release the right nostril and exhale through your right nostril. Inhale through the right nostril. Close right, release left, and then exhale through the left nostril. Continue back and forth for a minute or longer. Your breathing should be relaxed and rhythmic.

ALTERNATE NOSTRIL BREATHING II

Hold up your right hand. Fold down your index and middle fingers. (You will be using your thumb and ring finger to hold down nostrils.) If you find this too uncomfortable, just use your thumb and index fingers. Close off your left nostril with your fingers. Inhale through your right nostril for a count of four. Lift your fingers and close your right nostril with your thumb. Exhale to a count of eight. Try this for about a minute and then switch sides. Close off your right nostril with your thumb, inhaling through your left nostril for a count of four. Lift your thumb and close off your left nostril with your fingers. Exhale to a count of eight.

ALTERNATE NOSTRIL BREATHING III

This exercise helps to clear and calm the mind. [Note: Pregnant woman should check with their doctor before retaining the breath.] Close off your right nostril with your thumb, and inhale to a count of four. Close off your left nostril with your fingers, holding your breath for a count of sixteen. Lift your thumb, and exhale for a count of eight. Inhale to a count of four. Close and hold for a count of sixteen. With fingers up, exhale for a count of eight. Continue for four or more rounds, and then sit for a few moments, relaxing your body and mind.

HOW TO BEGIN

> *Praise and blame, gain and loss, pleasure and sorrow come and go like the wind. To be happy, rest like a giant tree, in the midst of them all.*
> —Buddha

It may be helpful to skim through the entire book first before trying to physically do each pose. Getting familiar with the poses first will make your practice smoother and more enjoyable.

Select a sturdy, armless, straight-back chair that allows you to put your feet flat on the floor. Wear comfortable clothing. You may choose to remove your shoes and socks. A quiet area, free from distractions, is ideal. Relaxing music may enhance your practice.

SITTING POSTURES

There are two ways to sit in your chair throughout your yoga practice. The first, Relaxing Posture, is meant for resting the body. The other is a Yogic Posture, from which you start a pose.

RELAXING POSTURE

Sit all the way back in your chair with your feet resting comfortably on the floor. Let your hands rest on your thighs, either palms up or down. Close your eyes or just allow your gaze to drop softly ahead of you.

HOW TO BEGIN

Use relaxing posture to rest during your practice or in between poses. Relaxing between postures helps you prepare for moving again.

YOGIC POSTURE

Begin each posture by sitting tall with your back away from the back of the chair. Lengthen through the spine with your chest out and abs in. Imagine that you are being lifted from the very top of your head up to the ceiling. Think of this as your working posture.

DRISHTI

Many yoga students wonder where they are supposed to look when they are in a pose. Yogis call the focus of the eyes during a pose or meditation a *drishti*. The famous yogi and founder of Ashtanga Yoga, Sri K. Pattabhi Jois, popularized drishti techniques. Think of your drishti as where you should gaze during a pose. In this book, we often suggest that you look upward, straight out over your fingertips or wherever the neck and head is comfortable, depending on the pose. You may also practice many poses with your eyes closed or softly focusing on the floor.

BREATHING AND RELAXING

Using your breath when working in the postures adds to the experience.
Keep in mind that relaxed muscles stretch. As you linger in a pose, try relaxing your body. With your exhale, sink deeper into the posture. Typically, you exhale to lower into a pose and inhale to rise out of, or release, a pose. Approach challenging poses with patience and care.

INTENTION

You can set an intention before you start each yoga session. This might be what you wish to accomplish, change, or feel as a result of your practice. It could also be a physical attribute, such as "I am going to feel more flexible after class today," or a mental or emotional intention, such as "I am going to stop worrying about things over which I have no control" or "I am going to have a softer heart with those I love." You might decide to dedicate your workout to someone who is on your mind.

Next, try to clear your mind of all busy thoughts. Leave the past behind, and try not to think ahead to the future. Focus on the present moment.

WARM-UP POSTURES

The warm-up is intended to move each joint through a comfortable range of motion and increase the blood flow in your muscles, preparing them for longer-held and more challenging postures.

Try to begin each posture with the following:
Sit tall, lengthening through the spine.
Keep shoulders neutral with chest raised.
Keep abdominal muscles engaged.
Plant feet firmly on the floor.
Relax the limbs and face.
Repeat each posture at least three times.

TORSO

1. CAT/COW
Rest your hands on your thighs. Exhale as you look to your navel, rounding your back and dropping your chin to your chest. Inhale and lengthen your spine, bending back slightly and pressing your chest and belly forward.

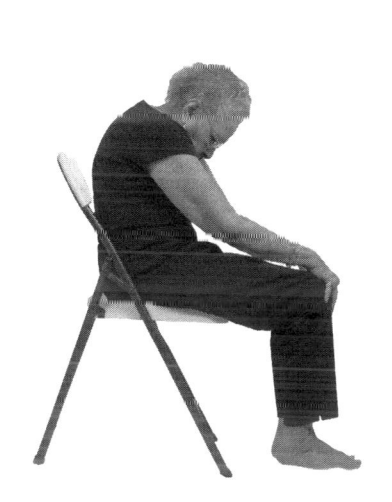

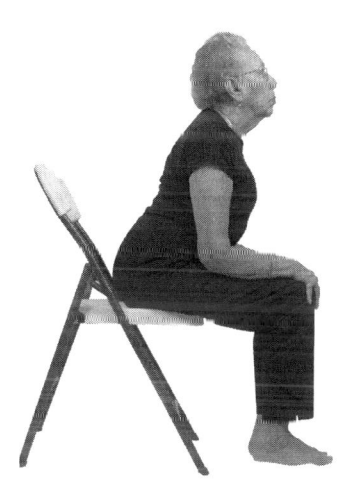

2. FLOWING AIRPLANE

Inhaling, reach your arms overhead. Exhale as you bring your chest forward toward your thighs, stretching your arms back behind you, parallel to the floor.

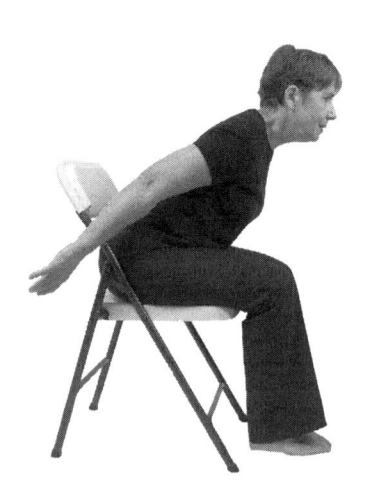

3. FLOWING SPINAL TWIST

Starting with your hands at your sides, inhale as you raise your arms overhead. Exhale as you turn to the right. Drop your left hand outside your right knee and hold the back of the chair by the seat with your right hand. Inhale as you raise your arms overhead and repeat on the left side.

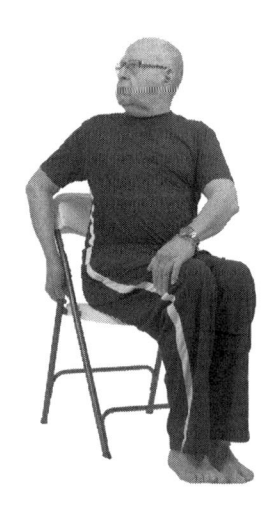

4. CIRCLING ARMS

Place your hands together at your heart center. Circle your arms out to your sides and overhead, bringing palms back together. Exhale as you lower your arms down to your heart center. After repeating three times, reverse directions.

Starting at your heart center, inhale as you raise your arms overhead, and then exhale as you circle down, bringing your hands to your heart center again. Repeat three times.

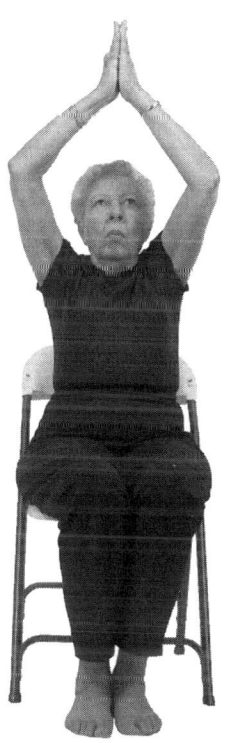

UPPER BODY

5. SHOULDER SHRUGS
Inhale as you lift your shoulders up high toward your ears. Exhale and drop your shoulders as low as you can.

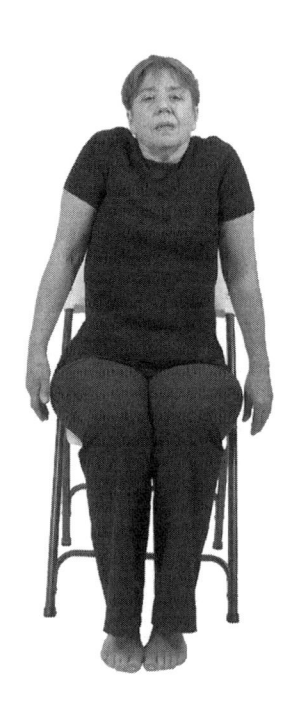

6. SHOULDER ROLLS
Breathe comfortably as you roll your shoulders in three circles forward and then in three circles backward.

7. SHOULDER RELEASE
Inhale and place your fingertips on your shoulders. Exhale and touch your elbows together in front of your body. Inhale and pull your elbows back as far as you can comfortably.

WARM-UP POSTURES

8. SIDE-TO-SIDE NECK WARM-UP
Inhale and turn your head to the right (as if trying to look over your shoulder). Exhale and turn your head back to center. Inhale and turn your head to the left. Exhale and turn your head back to center.

9. TURTLE NECK
Sitting tall, move your head straight forward, keeping your chin parallel to the floor. Then move your head back, centering it over the spine.

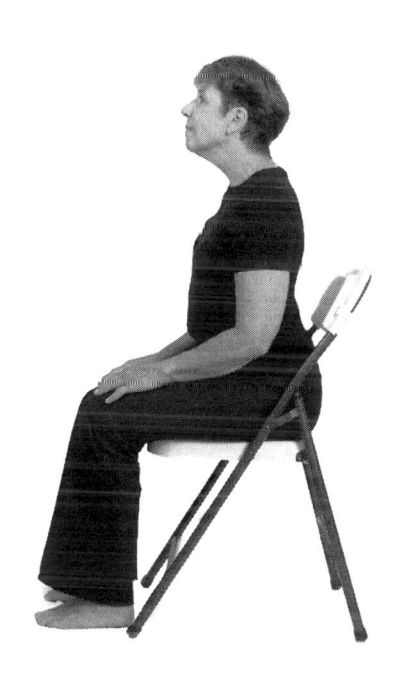

10. NECK PENDULUM
Inhale and sit up as tall as you can. Exhaling, gently drop your chin to your chest. Inhaling, roll your right ear to your right shoulder. Exhaling, drop your chin to your chest. Inhaling, roll your left ear to your left shoulder. Exhaling, drop your chin to your chest. Inhale and come back to center.

WARM-UP POSTURES

11. HALF MOON

Bring your arms overhead with your palms together. Inhale, stretch, and reach up as tall as you can. Exhale as you bend gently to the right. Inhale, stretch, and reach up tall. Exhale as you bend gently to the left. Inhale as you stretch tall again.

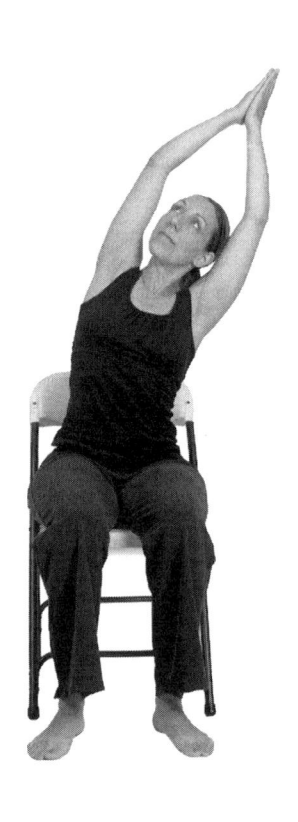

LOWER BODY

12. KNEE LIFTS

Sit tall with your hands at your side. Inhale and lift your right knee up. Exhale and lower your leg. Repeat four times and then switch to your left leg.

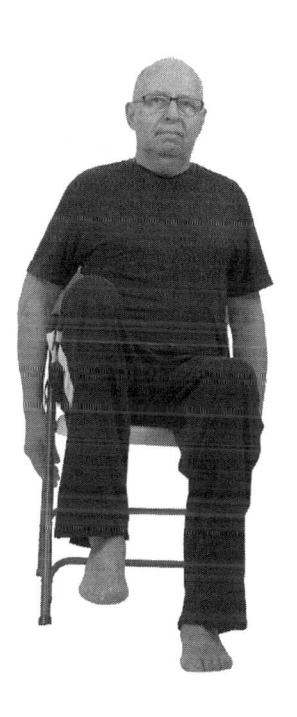

13. KNEE CROSS AND ROTATE

Inhale and lift your right knee up. Exhale and cross your right knee over your left leg. Inhale and lift your right knee back up. Exhale and uncross the knee, putting your foot down. Repeat four times and then switch to your left leg.

Inhale and lift your right knee up. Exhale, rotating your lifted knee to your right side. Inhale, moving your knee back to center and exhale your leg down. Repeat four times and then switch to your left leg.

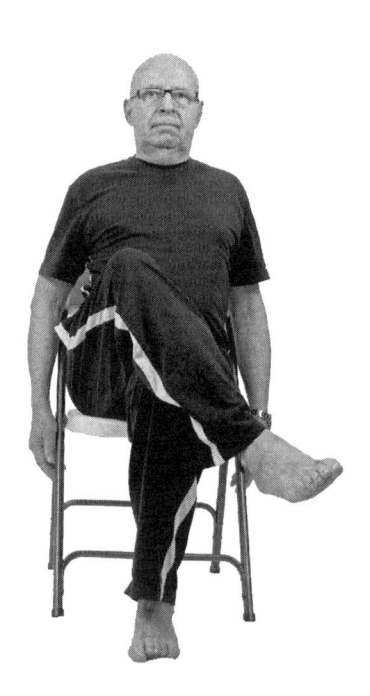

WARM-UP POSTURES

14. KNEE TO CHEST
Inhale your right knee to your chest and place your foot in the chair or hold your shin with your hands. Exhale. Inhale your chin to the ceiling. Exhale your chin to your chest. Breathe into your lower back, and then breathe into your middle back. Inhale into your shoulder blades, and exhale down your arms. Inhale your chin to the ceiling. Exhale as you lower your leg and relax your body. Repeat with your left leg.

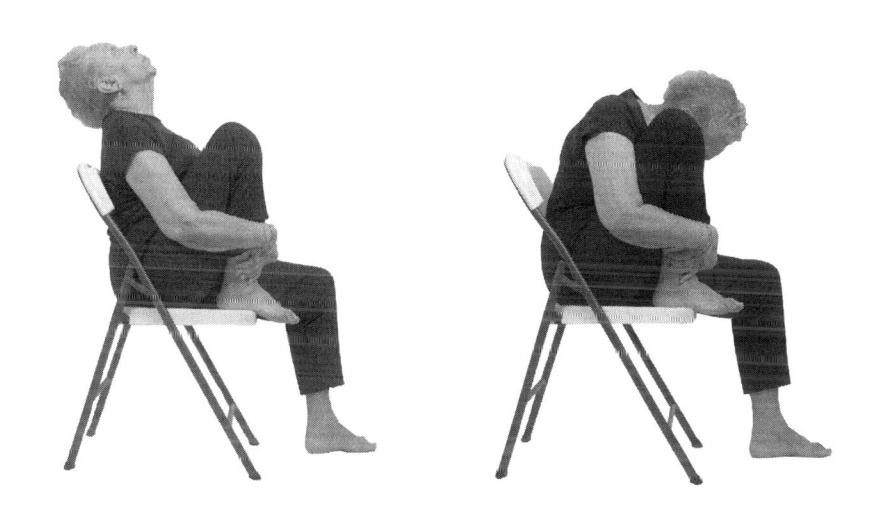

15. LEG EXTENSIONS
Inhale and lift one knee high, and then straighten your leg. Exhale and bend your knee, and then lower your foot to the floor. Repeat three to six times on each leg.

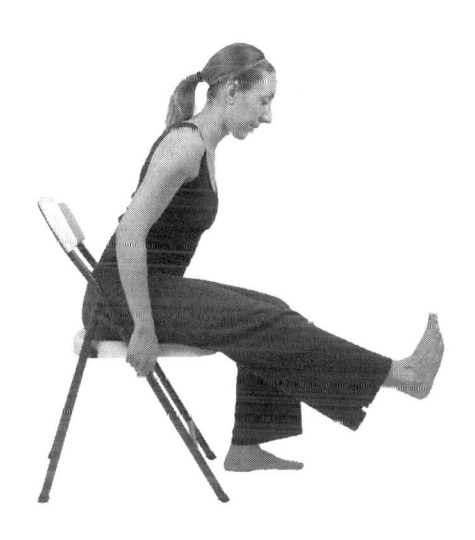

WARM-UP POSTURES

16. ANKLE ROTATIONS
Inhale both feet up until your legs are straight. Rotate your feet several times, and then reverse the rotation. Point and flex your feet several times. With your feet flexed, touch your toes together as your heels splay out, and then touch your heels together as your toes splay out. Repeat several times. End with several flutter kicks.

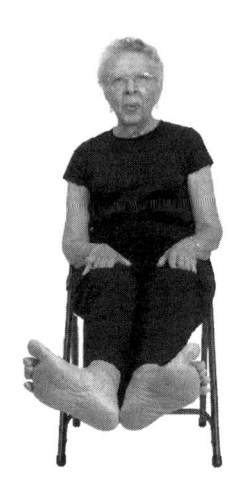

17. TOE AND HEEL TAPPING
With feet flat on the floor, challenge the left and right sides of the brain by tapping the heel of your left foot at the same time that you tap the toes of your right foot. Switch to right heel and left toes.

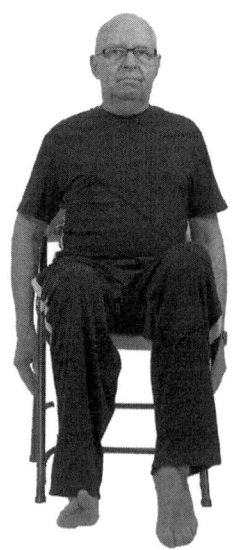

WARM-UP POSTURES

18. FOOT ROTATIONS
Start with feet flat on the floor, and then rise up on your toes. Roll around to the outside of your feet, back to your heels, and to the inside of your feet. Repeat several times, and then reverse directions.

19. FOOT PRESSES
With feet hip width apart, point toes toward the sky. Hold for a few seconds, then bring the toes down and lift both heels. Hold for a few seconds.

20. SUN SALUTATION
Use this sequence as a way to warm up. Take your knees apart slightly wider than hip width. Inhaling, sweep your arms out to your sides and overhead. Exhaling, place your hands on your thighs as you lean forward, flattening your back. Inhale and then exhale as you fold over, letting your hands rest on your shins or the floor. Inhale and come back up with a flat back, bringing your hands back to your thighs. Exhale as you sit back in your chair and relax.

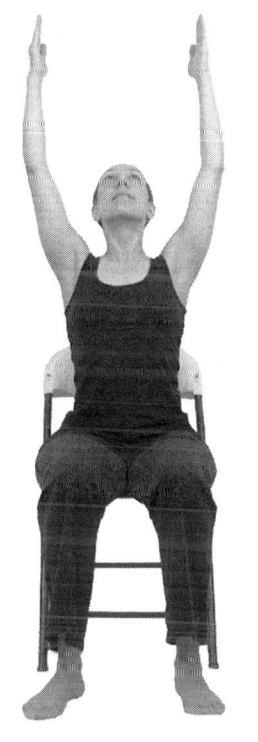

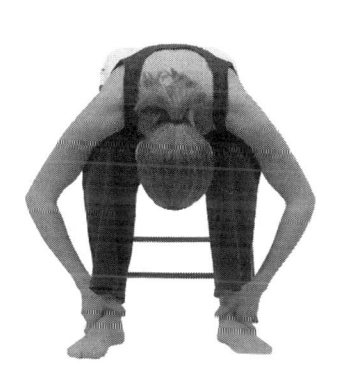

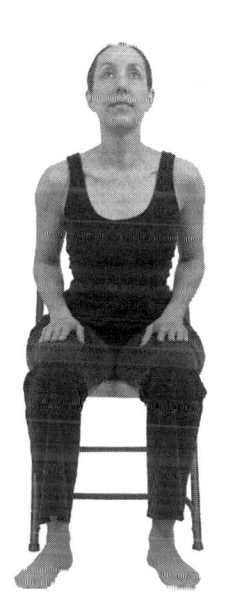

ENDURANCE AND STRENGTH POSTURES

> *When people are put into positions slightly above what they would expect to achieve, they're apt to excel.*
> —Richard Bronson

For all the postures below, sit toward the front of your chair. Take three to five breaths per exercise. Most importantly, do not hold your breath while doing any postures.

SEATED POSTURES

21. CHAIR POSE
Hold the sides of the chair as you stand halfway out of your seat. Let the hips and thighs hover above the seat of the chair. Take hands to prayer position or extend them out straight in front of the body. Hold for a couple of breaths, and then sit carefully back onto your chair.

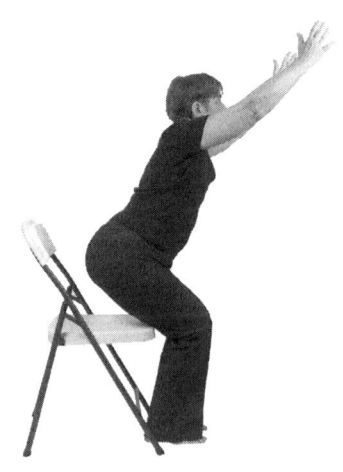

22. ARM CIRCLES

With arms out at your sides in a T-shape and palms facing the floor, slowly make small circles in a forward motion. Try to keep the shoulders down and relaxed. Start making the circles bigger. Without lowering the arms, switch directions, starting with small circles. After several breaths, make the circles bigger. Shake the arms gently after you bring them down to your sides.

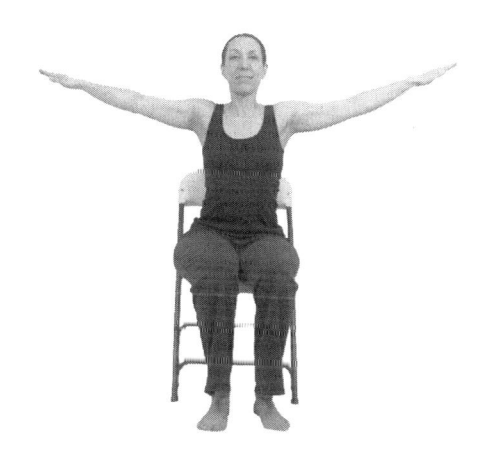

23. TRIANGLE

Sit up tall. Inhale and lift your right arm straight up beside your ear and let your left arm hang down by your side or gently grasp the side of the chair. Looking straight ahead, exhale over to the left. Hold for three or more breaths. Return to center and then switch to your left arm. Repeat at least twice.

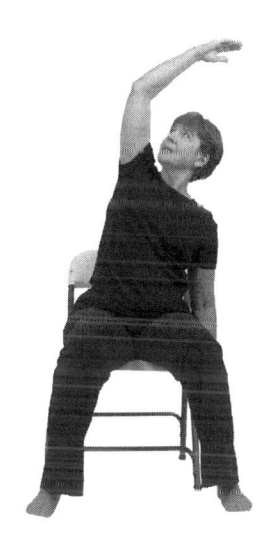

ENDURANCE AND STRENGTH POSTURES

24. PRAYER SQUAT FLOW

Plant feet firmly onto the floor with legs wide apart and toes pointing slightly outward. Inhaling, raise your arms out to your sides, then overhead, crossing your arms. Exhaling, lean forward, letting your arms sweep down and out to the sides, then to the space between your knees, with hands briefly crossing. Inhaling, sweep arms out and up in a circling motion overhead. Continue to flow up and down for as many rounds as you like.

Variation: Keep your torso more upright throughout the flow.

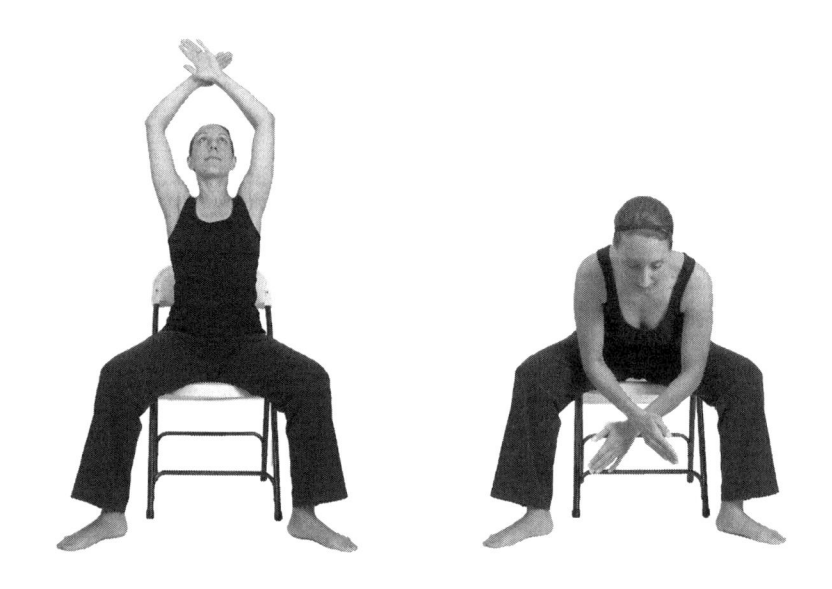

25. ELBOW TO KNEE

Inhale and place your fingertips on your shoulders. Exhale and move your left elbow down to your right knee. Inhale up to your starting position. Exhale and move your right elbow to your left knee. Inhale and return to your starting position. Repeat several times.

Variation: Raise your knee as you exhale your elbow to your knee.

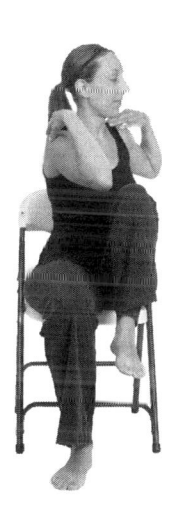

26. REVOLVED TRIANGLE

Sit tall with your feet wide apart. Place your right hand on your left knee as you lean slightly forward. Turn to the left and place your left hand on your hip. Hold for two or three breaths. Turn to the right and repeat.

Variation: For a deeper stretch, exhale as you slide your right hand down the left leg as low as possible.

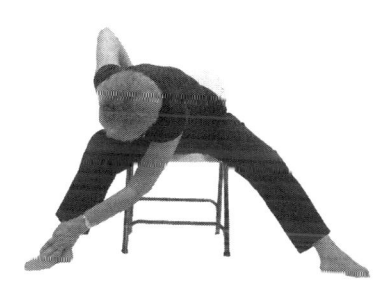

ENDURANCE AND STRENGTH POSTURES

Note: We describe the Warrior Poses in order from Warrior I, to Warrior II, to Reverse Warrior, and then to Side Angle. These poses flow nicely together. Once you become comfortable with the Warriors, try practicing them in various orders.

27. WARRIOR I
Spread your legs wide apart. Turn to your right, pushing your left leg back and pressing the ball of your foot onto the floor. Straighten your left leg as much as possible. Raise both arms up, aiming your fingers and gaze to where the ceiling meets the wall, or higher. Hold for a few breaths.
Variation: Turn your palms up.

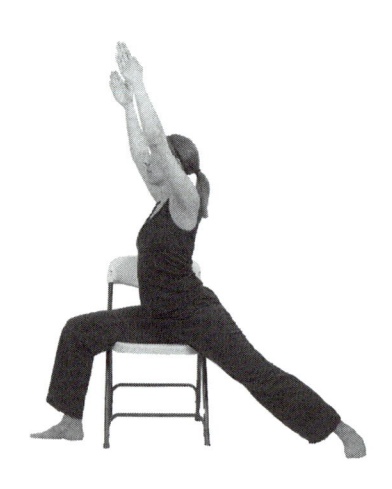

28. WARRIOR II
Starting from Warrior I, turn your torso, allowing the hips and shoulders to face forward. Bring both arms down to shoulder height with your palms down. Let your toes point slightly to your right, and then press the outside edge of your left foot onto the floor. Look just past the fingertips on your right hand. Try to relax your shoulders and keep them square. Hold for a few breaths.

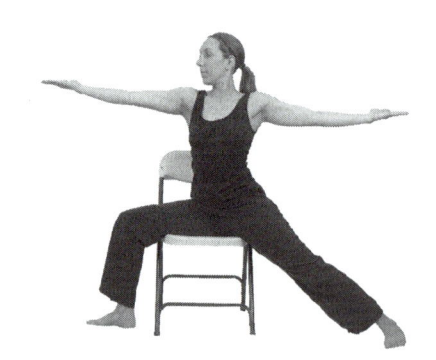

ENDURANCE AND STRENGTH POSTURES

29. REVERSED WARRIOR
Starting from Warrior II, allow your left hand to rest on your left hip or your left leg while reaching your right hand toward the ceiling. Look toward your right hand. Hold for a few breaths.

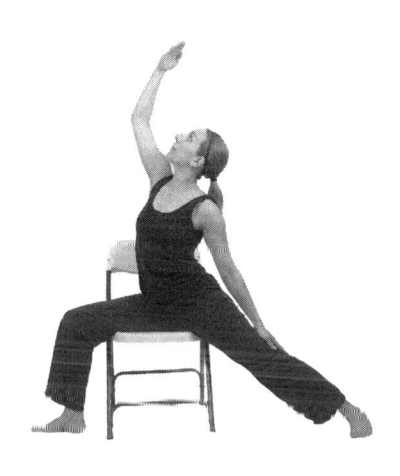

30. SIDE-ANGLE WARRIOR
Starting from Reverse Warrior, lean to your right, resting your right arm on your right thigh. Inhale your left arm overhead. Gently press your left shoulder back. Look toward your left hand. Hold for a few breaths. Variation: Keep your left hand on your hip.

Turn back to center. Repeat all of the Warrior postures on your left side.

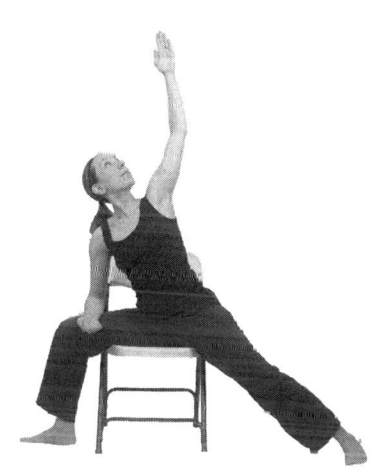

31. CAMEL

Place your palms against your lower back on each side of your spine. Expand your chest, lifting your chin slightly. Press elbows toward one another. Hold for a few breaths and then release.

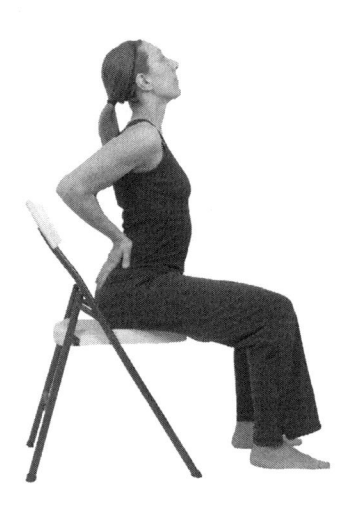

32. GATE

Extend the left leg directly out to the side. Place your left hand lightly on your left thigh. Inhale and lift your right arm up toward the ceiling. Exhale and gently bend from the waist toward the left. Repeat on the other side.

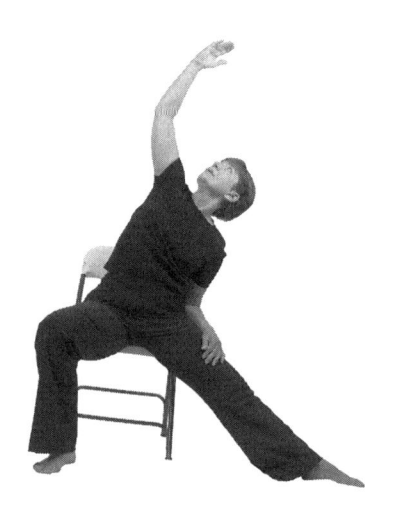

33. EAGLE

Cross your right leg over the left, trying to lock your right toes behind your left leg. Spread the arms wide and then cross them in front of the body to make an X by crossing the left arm on top of the right so that your elbows are stacked one on top of the other. Continue to wrap the forearms so that the palms and fingers of each hand face one another, or so that the backs of your hands touch. If this is not comfortable, just place your right hand on your left shoulder and your left hand on your right shoulder, giving yourself a hug. Repeat on the other side.

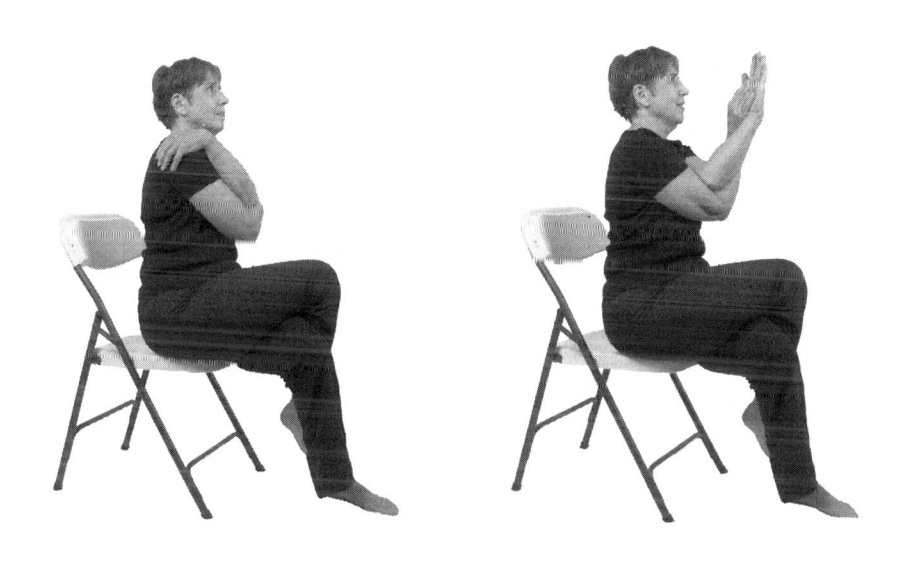

34. CHEST EXPANSION

Position feet hip width apart on the floor. Reach your arms behind you to grasp the chair back. Inhale and gently bring your chest forward until you feel a nice stretch in the front of your shoulders and chest.

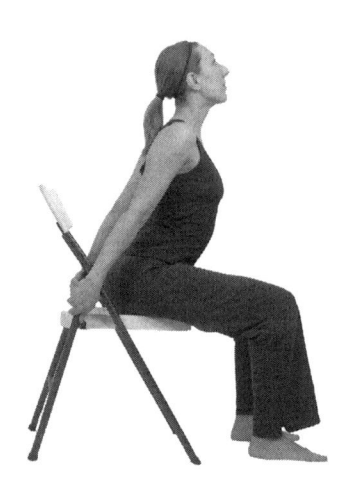

35. SPINAL TWIST

Let both legs turn to the right so that the left side of your body faces the middle of the room. Place your right hand on the right side of your seat back and the left on the left side. Gently look toward your right shoulder. Allow your exhales to help you twist slightly deeper. Hold for five to seven breaths and then switch sides.

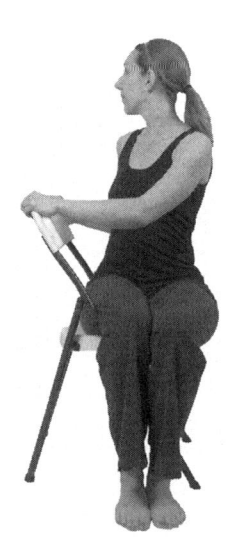

STANDING POSTURES

> *Health is wealth, Peace of mind is happiness, Yoga shows the way.*
> —Swami Vishnu-devananda

36. MOUNTAIN POSE (the foundation of all standing poses)

Like many other poses, those that appear to be "easy" or "simple" often provide great opportunity for deep, focused physical and mental work. Try the simple version of Mountain below and then use some of the bulleted tips for future practices. Stand tall with your feet about hip distance apart and your arms at your sides, slightly away from your body. Keep your chest high, abs in, and shoulders back and relaxed. Lift and spread your toes and the balls of your feet, and then lay them softly down on the floor. Rock back and forth and from side to side. Gradually reduce this swaying to a standstill, with your weight balanced evenly on your feet.

- Put a tiny bend in your knees and see if you feel your back and abdominal muscles work even harder.
- Lengthen your spine, reaching the crown of your head toward the sky while keeping your shoulders back and down.
- Imagine three points on the bottom of each foot—one on the heel and the other two on each side of the ball of the foot. Root these six points down, keeping the natural arches in your feet.

STANDING POSTURES

- Slightly or completely close your eyes to challenge your balance. Build confidence in this balance as you think about what it feels like to be a mountain.
- Visualize electrically charged roots moving down from the bottom of the feet and fingertips into the Earth and from the crown of the head upward.

Variation: Walk around your chair several times while engaging the principles of Mountain Pose. A little walk in Mountain Pose may help you be more aware of your walking posture.

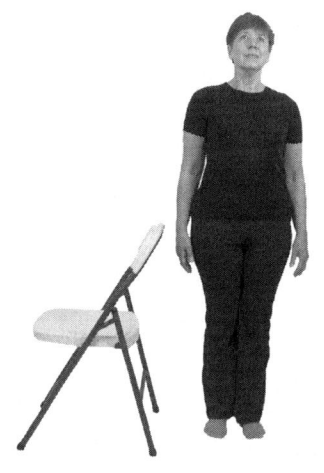

37. CAT/COW

Bend your knees, getting into a semi-squat position. Place your hands on your thighs just above your knees. Exhale as you look to your navel and round your back like a scared cat. Inhale as you look up, pressing your tailbone out and your chest forward, swaying your back. Repeat several times in a flowing manner.

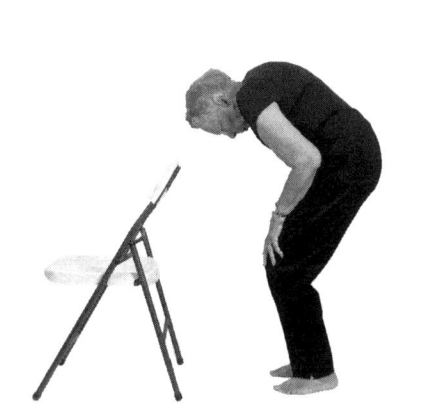

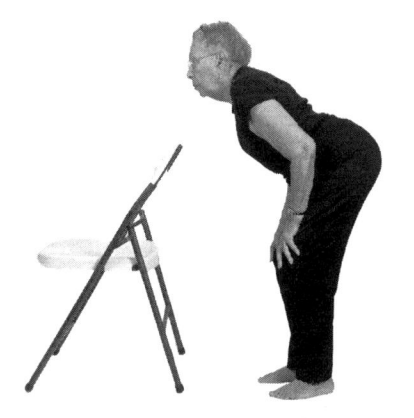

38. ARM CIRCLES

With arms out in a T-shape and palms facing the floor, slowly make small circles in a forward motion. Try to keep the shoulders down and relaxed as you start making the circles bigger. Without lowering the arms, switch directions, starting with small circles. After several breaths, make the circles bigger. Shake your arms gently after you bring them down to your sides.

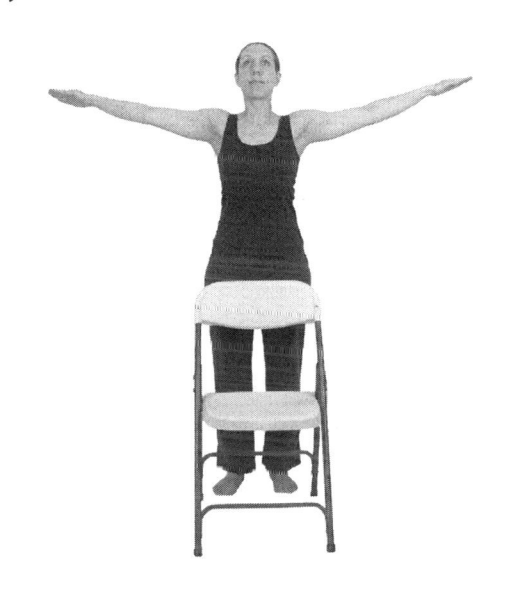

39. PRAYER SQUAT FLOW

Plant feet firmly onto floor with legs wide apart and toes pointed slightly outward. Inhaling, raise your arms out to the sides and then overhead. Exhaling, bend your knees into a wide-legged squat and lean forward, letting your arms sweep down and out to your sides, then to the space between your knees, with hands crossing. Inhaling, sweep your arms out and up in a circling motion overhead as you straighten your legs. Continue this flow for as many rounds as you like.

Variation: Keep your torso more upright throughout the flow. To challenge your balance, try closing your eyes for a few rounds.

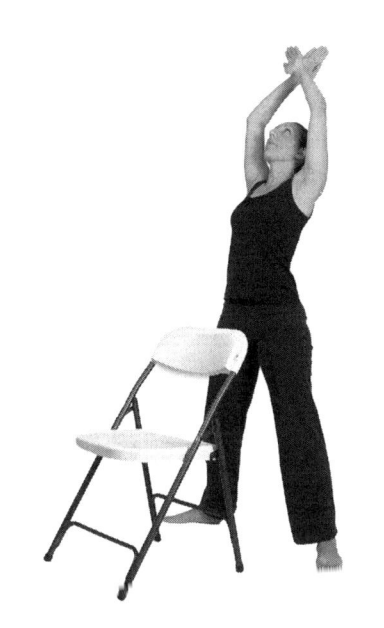

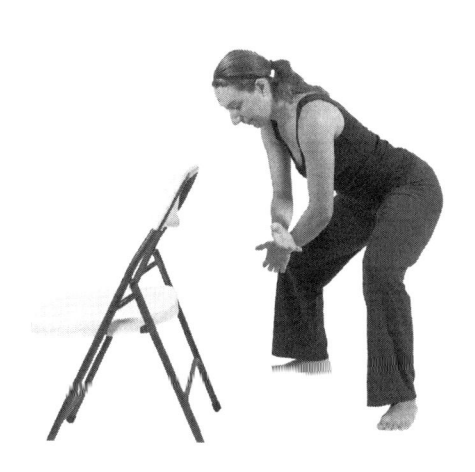

STANDING POSTURES

40. HALF MOON
Bring your arms overhead with your palms together. Inhale as you stretch up as tall as you can. Exhaling, bend gently to the right. Inhaling, return to center. Exhaling, bend gently to the left. Inhaling, return to center. Repeat two or three times, and then rest your arms at your sides.

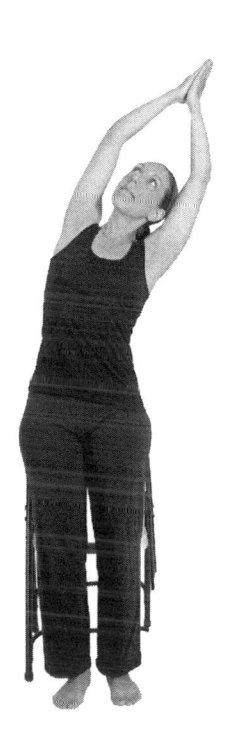

41. TRIANGLE

Starting from Mountain Pose, separate your feet at least two feet apart, making them parallel. Inhale your left arm up beside your left ear. Exhale and bend to your right side, allowing your right hand to slide down your leg. Avoid bending forward, and keep your hips squared. Hold for three or more breaths. Return to center, and then switch to your right. Repeat at least twice.

Variation: With feet at least two feet apart, point your left foot to the left, and rotate your right heel slightly to the right. Inhale as you lift your arms up in a T-position. Exhale as you lower your right hand down your right leg, either above or below your knee, and your left hand up to the sky. Keep your left shoulder back, and avoid bending forward. Try to keep both sides of your body lengthened. Repeat on the right side.

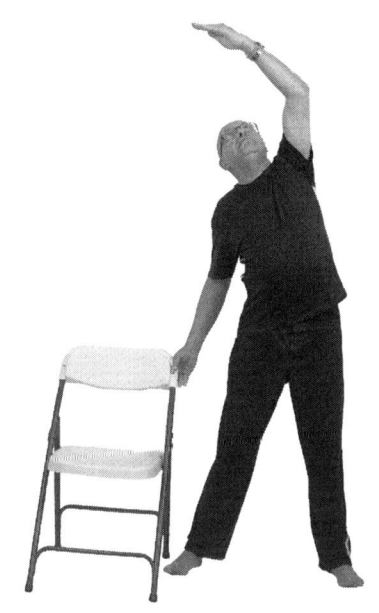

STANDING POSTURES

42. REVOLVED TRIANGLE

Starting from Mountain Pose, separate your feet wider than shoulder width apart, with both feet facing forward. Raise your arms to shoulder height in a T-position. Turn to the right, bend from the hip, and exhale down, bringing your left hand to your right leg, as low as possible, with both legs straight. Hold for three or more breaths. Inhale up. Turn to the left and repeat.

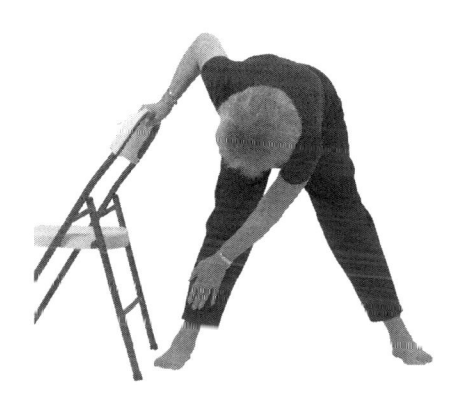

43. WARRIOR I

Stand behind your chair. Take your feet into a stance at least two feet apart. Point your right foot to the right, and rotate your left heel slightly to the left. Turn your torso to the right, and bend your right knee slightly. Inhale and bring both arms straight up (or just the right arm if you are holding onto the chair back), aiming your fingers and gaze to where the ceiling and wall meet, or higher. Hold for a few breaths.

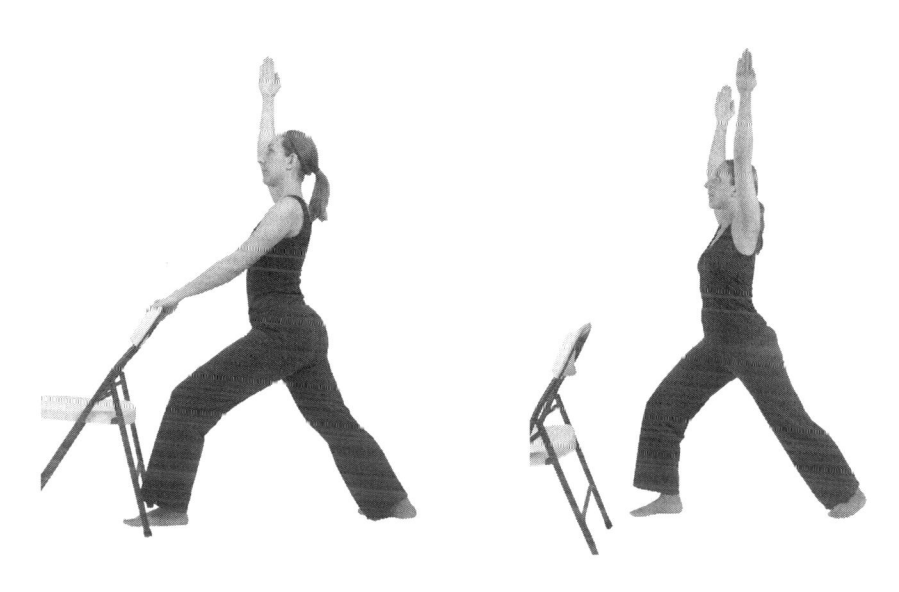

44. WARRIOR II

Starting from Warrior I, turn your torso to the front, bringing one or both arms down to shoulder height, with the palms down. Look just over your right fingertips. Try to relax your shoulders and square them to the front. Hold for a few breaths.

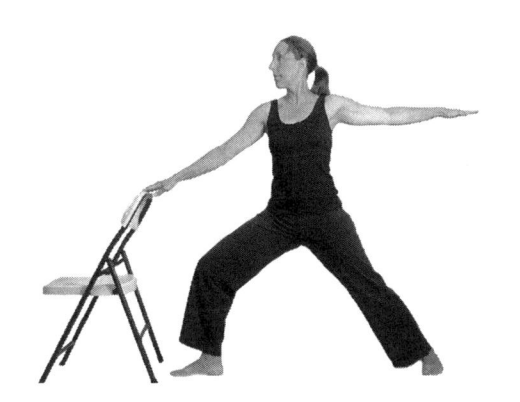

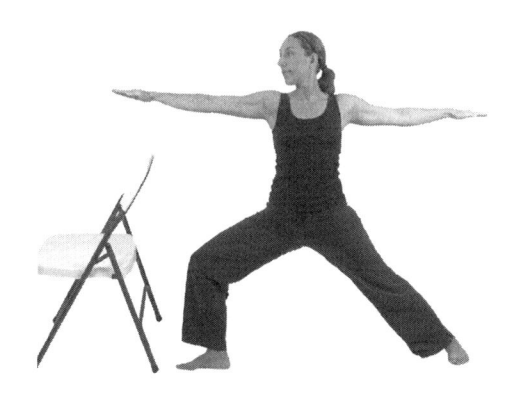

45. REVERSED WARRIOR

Starting from Warrior II, allow your left hand to rest on your left hip or leg. Rotate your right palm up, and then reach your right hand toward the ceiling. Keep your gaze upward toward your hand. Hold for a few breaths.

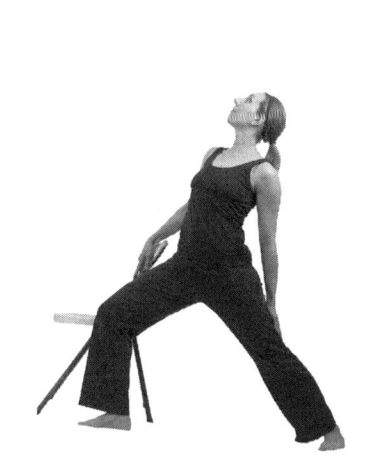

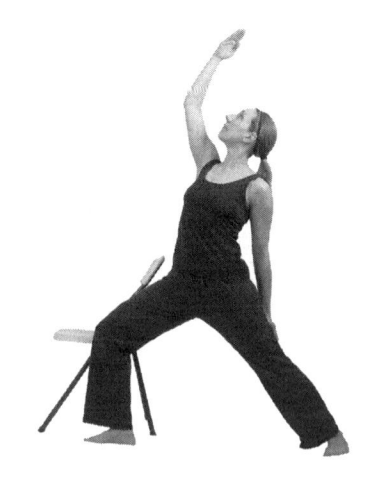

46. SIDE-ANGLE WARRIOR

Starting from Reverse Warrior, lean over and rest your right arm on your right thigh. Inhale your left arm straight overhead. Look toward your left hand. Hold for a few breaths.

Turn back to center. Repeat all of the Warrior postures on your left side.

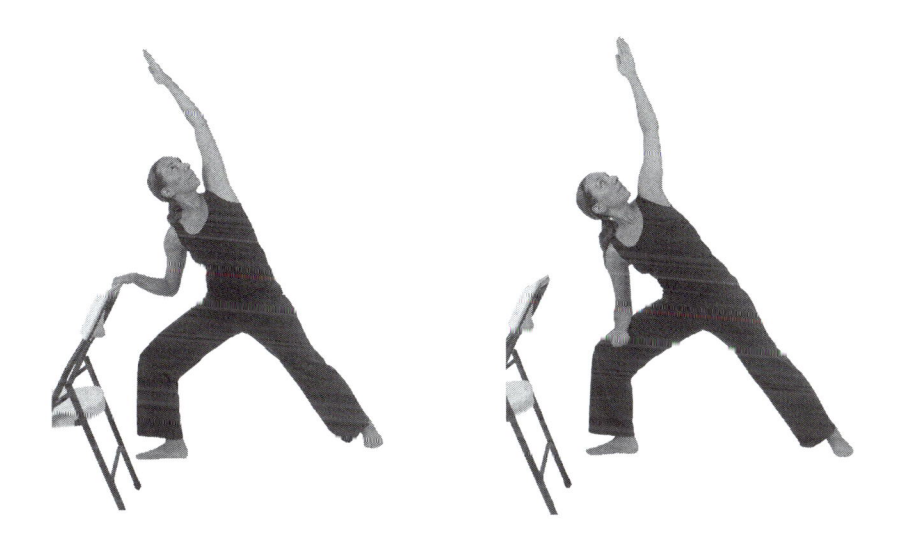

47. CAMEL

Stand with feet about hip width apart. Place your palms against your lower back on each side of your spine. Expand your chest, lifting your chin slightly. Press elbows toward one another. Hold for a few breaths and then release.

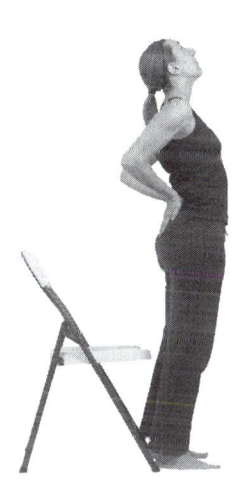

48. DOWNDOG

Downdog is a staple pose for many yoga classes. Starting behind your chair, grasp the chair back. Step back until your hips are stacked over your feet. Think of yourself as if you are an upside-down L or 90-degree angle. Your arms should be straight out from your shoulders. Enjoy stretching through your shoulders and the backs of your legs. Try to flatten the back as much as possible, and bring your head between your upper arms.

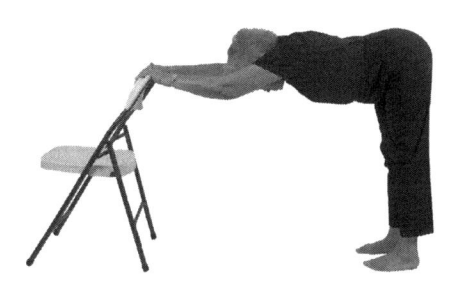

49. LEG RAISE

Stand behind your chair. Place one hand on the chair back for balance, if necessary. Slowly inhale your right leg to the side. Hold for two to three breaths, and then slowly exhale your leg down. Repeat the exercise about four times for each leg. Now try the exercise with your leg extending behind you (four times for each leg). Then step to the side of your chair, extending your leg to the front (again, four times for each leg). Remember to keep your leg straight and the knee soft.

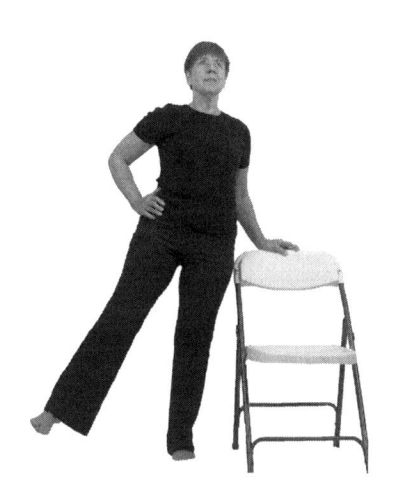

50. FORWARD BEND

In one variation, you stretch more through your back and spine, and in the other, you stretch more through your hamstrings.

For the back and spine:
Stand up tall with your feet together. Inhale your arms straight up to the ceiling. Exhale and slowly bend forward from your hips, letting your arms move out to your sides as you move toward the floor. Bend your knees so your hands can reach the floor. Allow your torso to rest on your thighs. Let your spine elongate and stretch.

For the hamstrings:
Stand up tall with your feet together. Inhale your arms straight up to the ceiling. Exhale and slowly bend forward from your hips. Sweep your arms across the ceiling and down the wall. Keep your legs straight, but avoid locking your knees. Allow your arms to fall loose, with the top of your head facing the floor. Breathe naturally, allowing your body to lower a little more with each exhale. Slowly roll up to a standing posture.

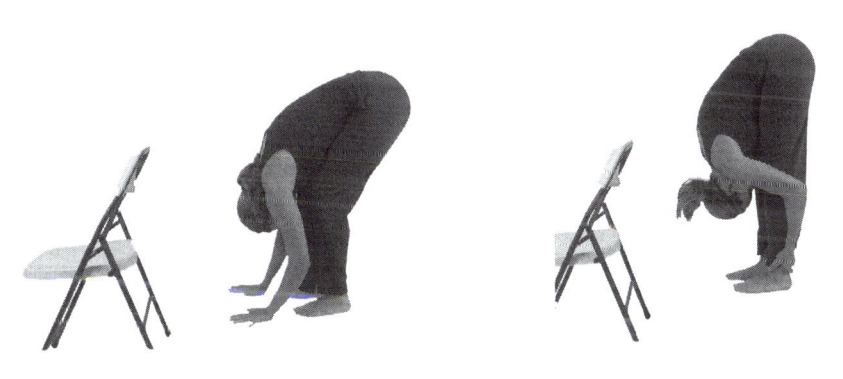

BALANCE POSTURES

> *We don't know who we are until we see what we can do.*
> —Martha Grimes

Practice balance because it is your best defense against a fall. Keep in mind that you do simple balance every time you take a step. You <u>only</u> need the chair to get into some balancing postures. Hold the chair to begin, and then let go once you are in the pose. If you feel unsteady when balancing on one leg, put your other foot down. Reaching for a chair is not advised. It is unlikely that a chair will be handy when you need one, but your foot is always with you. In our teaching experience, we found that when you make a habit of putting your foot down instead of depending on a chair, you are much safer from a fall.

For balance postures, it helps to relax the body and focus your eyes on something that does not move.

BALANCE POSTURES

51. BALANCE ON TOES
Rise up gently on your toes. Bring hands to your heart center and then overhead, with your palms together. Hold for three or four breaths.

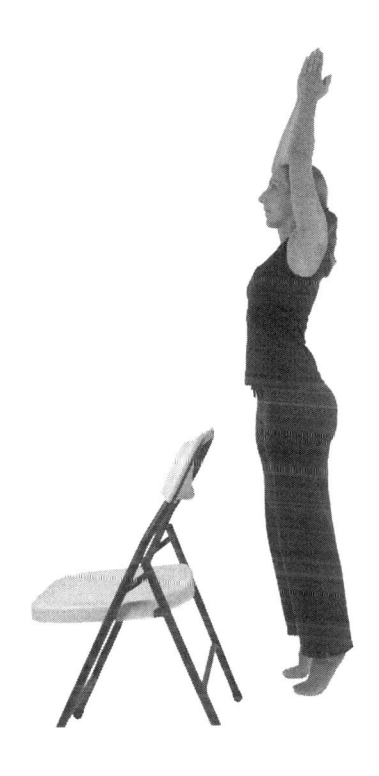

52. FLAMINGO
Alternate picking up your right and left foot several times. Increase the length of time you hold your balance.

53. KNEE LIFTS
Bring your right knee up in front, straighten your leg, bend again, and put it down. Repeat with your left knee.

BALANCE POSTURES

54. KNEE TO CHEST
Bring your right knee up in front, hold onto your shin, and gently pull your knee into your chest. Hold for three or four breaths. Repeat with your left knee.

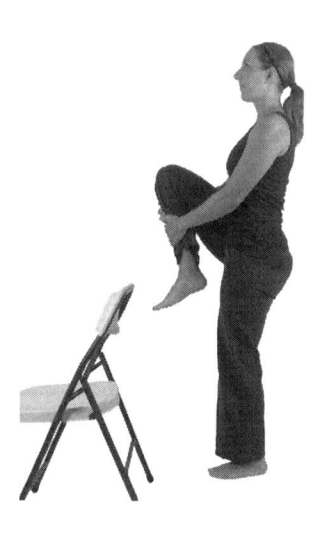

55. KNEE UP TWIST
Stand beside your chair. Inhale your left knee up, and extend your arms out in a T-shape. Turn to the left, bringing your left hand to the back and your right hand to the front. Hold for a few breaths. Try looking toward your left hand. Repeat on the other side.

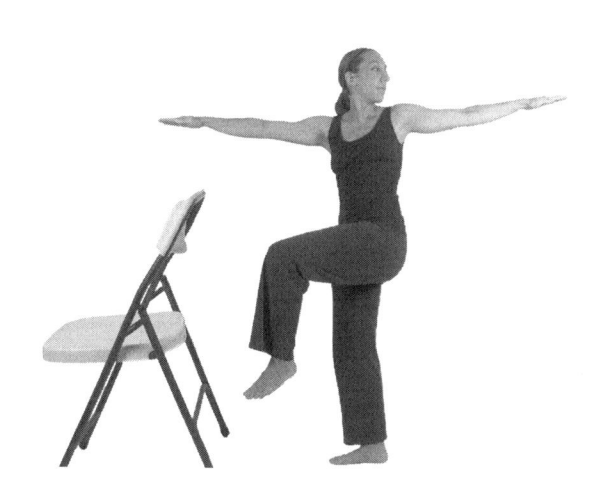

56. TREE

Standing tall, extend your right leg to the side, with your toe touching the floor. Slide your heel to your left ankle. Raise your foot up to the calf or thigh, keeping the knee pressed to the side. Avoid putting the foot by the knee. You might have your arms in T-position, hands at your heart center, or overhead. Hold the posture for a few breaths, and then repeat on the left.

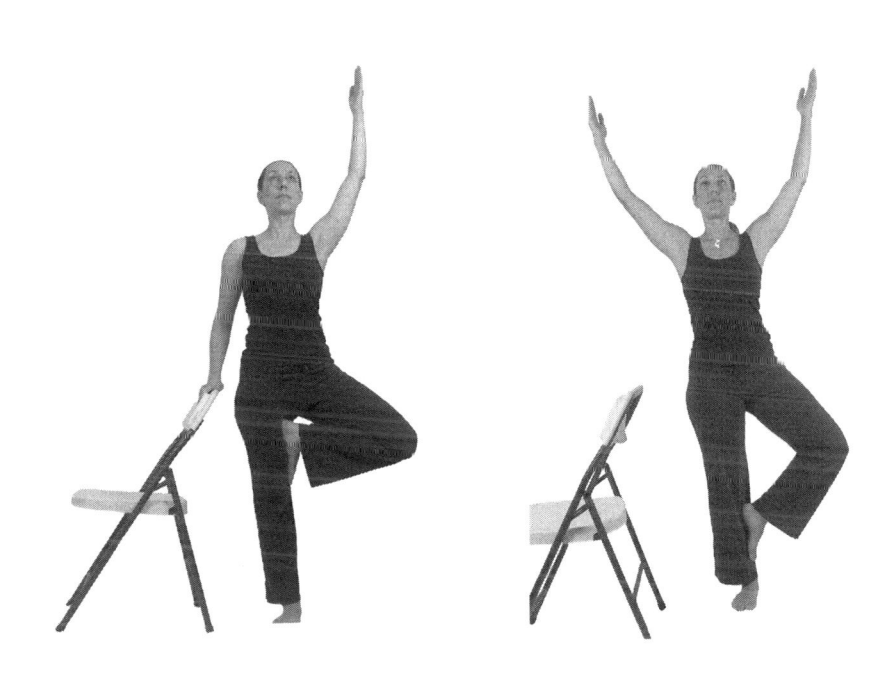

BALANCE POSTURES

57. DANCER'S POSE
Stand tall. Hold the back of the chair with your left hand. If needed, bend your right knee and grasp your right ankle with your right hand. When you feel in balance, inhale the left hand to the ceiling. Repeat on the other side.

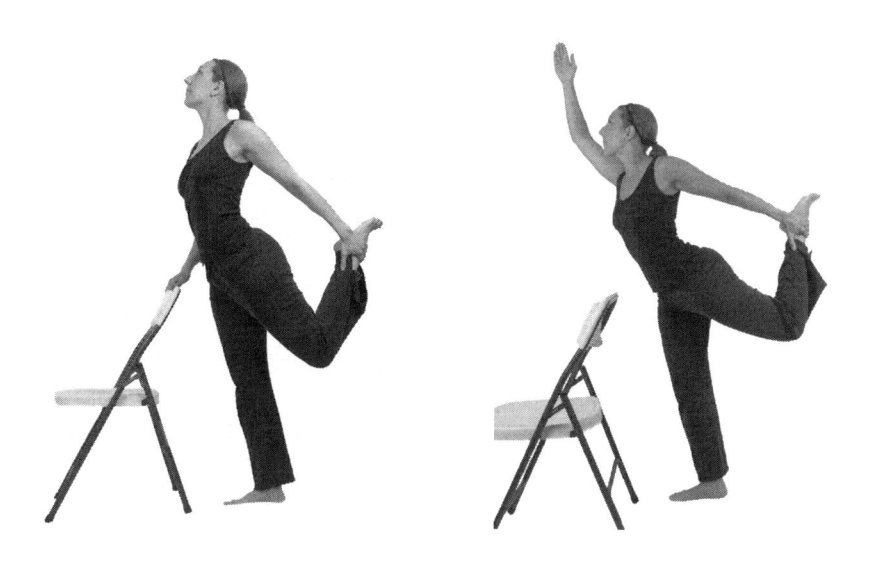

58. DANCER WITH HALF BOW
Starting from Dancer's Pose, gently push your foot away from your body into a bow, then start leaning forward until your knee and head are close to level with the chair back. Repeat on the other side.

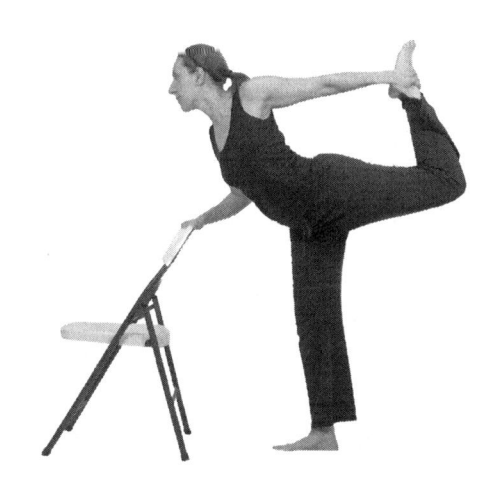

BALANCE POSTURES

59. WARRIOR III

Standing beside your chair, hold the chair back with your right hand, if needed. Keep the chair at arm's length. Stretch your left hand out making a half T-shape. Lean forward as you raise your right leg until your body is parallel to the floor. When you feel confident, bring your left hand out to complete the T and balance. Repeat on the other side.

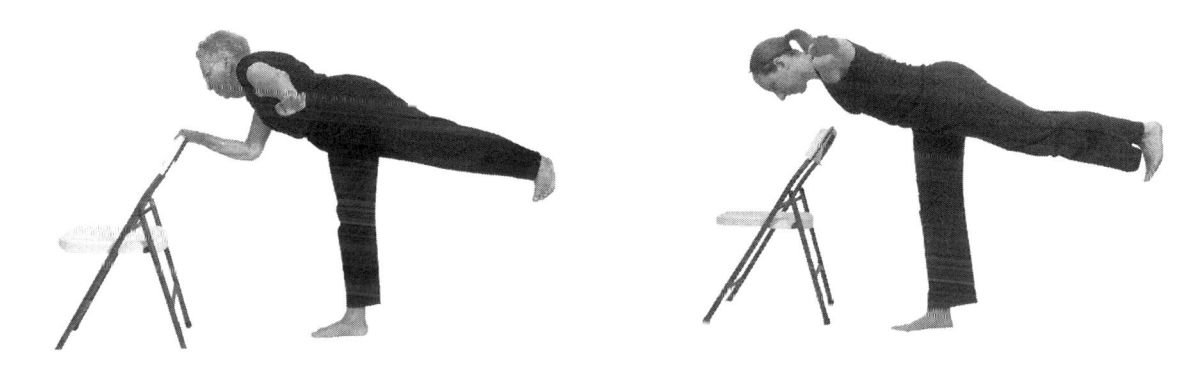

60. CHAIR SQUAT

Reach your arms straight out in front of you, bend your knees, and lower your hips as if you are sitting down onto a chair. Hold the posture for a few breaths. Now rise up on your toes and hold for a few breaths.

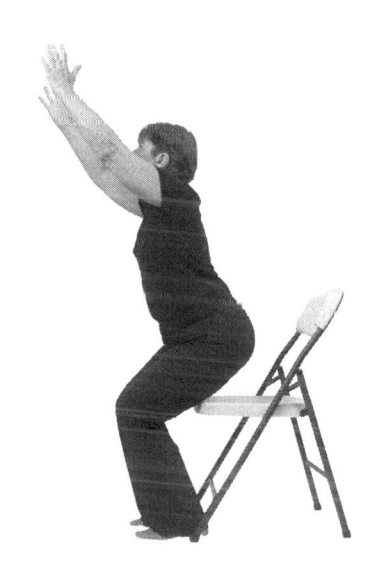

BALANCE POSTURES

61. CHAIR SQUAT ON ONE LEG
Place your right ankle just above your left knee. Reach your arms straight out in front of you or bring your hands to heart center in prayer position while bending your knees and lowering your hips as if you are sitting down onto a chair. Hold this posture for a few breaths. Repeat on your other leg.

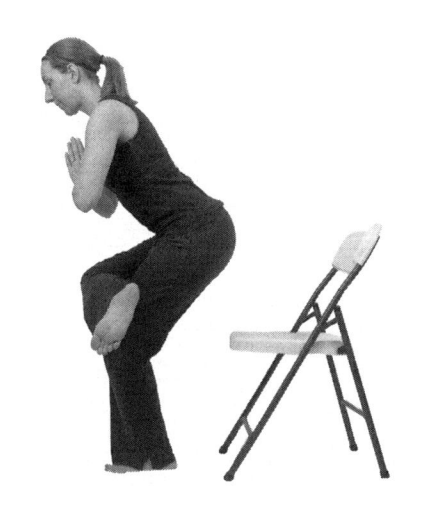

COOL-DOWN POSTURES

The purpose of a cool-down is to return your body to its resting state.

62. BACK OF SHOULDER STRETCH
Bring your right arm across your chest. Place your left hand or arm above or below your right elbow. Gently hug your right arm close to your chest. Repeat on the other side.

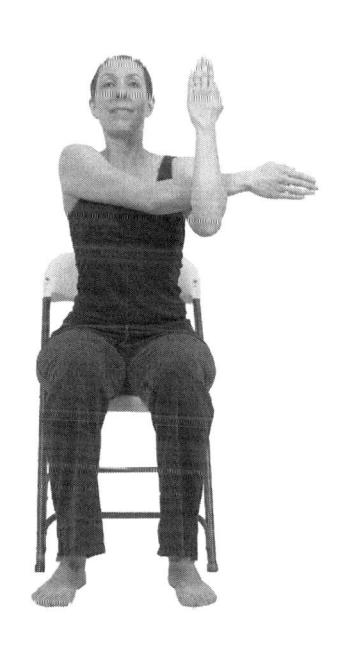

COOL-DOWN POSTURES

63. MIDDLE OF BACK STRETCH

Bring your hands in front of your chest, interlacing fingers, so that you are looking at your palms. Reach your hands as far away as is comfortable, bringing your chin toward your chest. Gently round your back

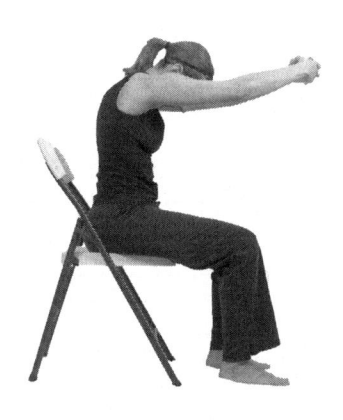

64. ROCK THE BABY

Sit tall and place your right ankle on your left thigh. Flex the right foot and hold it with your left hand while holding your knee with the right hand. Swing your foot back and forth as if you are rocking a baby, and then draw the leg in toward your chest as if you are hugging the baby. Repeat with your other leg.

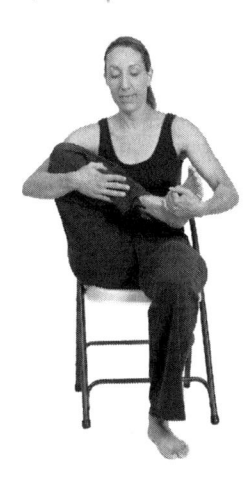

COOL-DOWN POSTURES

65. PIGEON

Sit tall and place your right ankle just above your left knee. Exhaling, bend forward from your hips, keeping your back flat. Hold for a few breaths. Inhaling, rise up into your Yogic Posture. Repeat on the other side.

If placing your ankle over your knee is difficult, sit forward in the chair, straighten your left leg and cross your right ankle over the left ankle, and then lean forward.

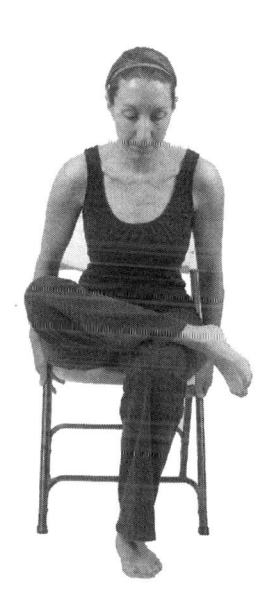

66. HAMSTRING STRETCH

Sit at the front edge of the chair and extend your right leg so it is almost straight (keep a slight bend in your knee). Your left foot should remain flat on the floor. Gently lean forward from your hips until you feel a stretch in the back of your right thigh. For a calf stretch, stay in this position, but do not lean forward. Keep the right heel on the floor and pull your toes up toward your shins as much as possible.

COOL-DOWN POSTURES

67. INNER THIGH STRETCH
Sit to the front edge of the chair. Bring your feet and knees wide apart. Place hands on the inside of each thigh, gently pressing outward. Exhale forward, hinging from the hips and keeping a flat back. Lower as much as you like, and then inhale up. Repeat a few times.

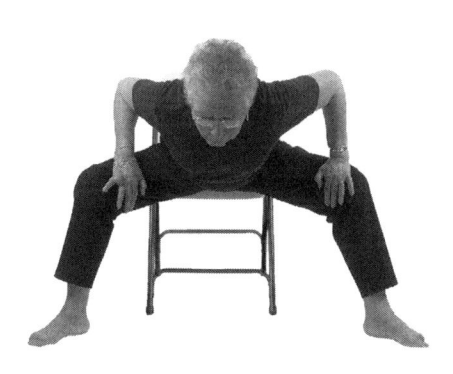

68. WRIST RELEASE
Holding your arms in front of the body, circle hands at the wrists several times in each direction. Now point and flex the hands a few times and release.

69. FACIAL RELEASE
While relaxing the rest of your body, close your eyes and scrunch up the nose, forehead, lips, and eyes. Inhale as the tension builds. Exhale as you release and stretch your face back out, opening your mouth and moving your jaw gently back and forth.

COOL-DOWN POSTURES

70. LION POSE
With palms down over your knees, take a deep breath. As you exhale, open your eyes wide and stick your tongue far out of your mouth, expelling breath with a throaty whisper. Repeat two times.

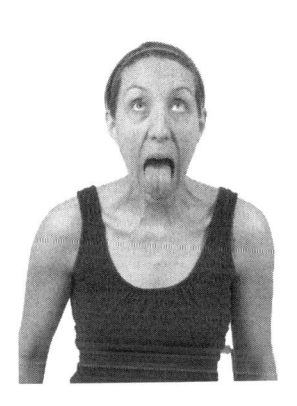

71. SEATED FORWARD BEND
Sitting tall, inhale your arms overhead. Exhale as you bend forward until you are relaxing with your chest on your lap and your arms dangling toward the floor. Remain here for a few breaths. Inhale as you slowly roll up one vertebra at a time: lower back, middle back, upper back, shoulder blades, shoulders, and head. Exhale to relax your body. Inhale and stretch out your arms and legs. Exhale and relax your body.

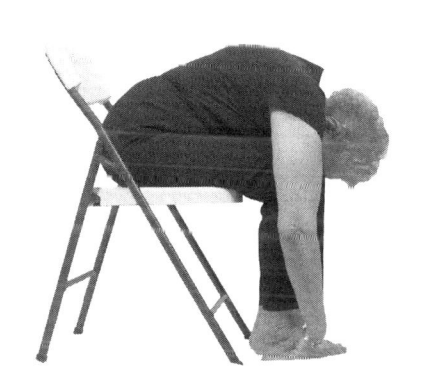

FINGER EXERCISES

Finger exercises are particularly good for arthritic finger joints.

72. FINGER FLEX
Stretch your fingers wide. Squeeze your fingertips down to the top pad of your hand, and then make a fist. Repeat twice.

73. FINGER SQUEEZE
Stretch your fingers wide. Beginning with your little fingers, bend each finger and push it into the top pad of your hand with your thumb.

74. FINGER STRETCHES
With your palm facing up, use other hand to gently pull each finger back one at a time toward the back of your hand; do not stretch thumb joint.

75. PULL AND TWIST
Starting with the little finger of your right hand, pull on your finger with your left hand, and then twist your finger away from you. Repeat on each of the other fingers.

76. JOINING
Place both hands down above your knees, with your thumb to the inside and your fingers to the outside. One at a time, bring each finger in to meet your thumb. Take each finger out again.

77. PARTING
Stretch your arms out in front of you, placing your palms together. Separate each finger, beginning with your little finger. Repeat twice.

78. THUMB TO FINGERS
Stretch the fingers out. Touch the base of your little fingers with your thumbs, and then slide your thumb out to the tip of your fingers. Repeat on each finger a few times.

FOOT AND TOE EXERCISES

Your feet will thank you for giving them a little attention.

Begin with your right foot just above your left knee. After completing all of the following steps with the right foot, switch to the left foot.

79. PULL AND TWIST
Starting with your little toe, pull and twist each toe away from you.

80. MASSAGE
Pound on the sole of your foot with your left fist. Massage the ball of your foot with both thumbs.

81. CLASP
Place the palm of your left hand on the ball of your foot and lace your fingers through your toes.

EYE EXERCISES

Eye exercises strengthen the extraocular muscles of the eyes and reduce tension. Keep your head and torso still while doing these exercises.

82. UP-DOWN RIGHT-LEFT
Look up and look down three times, close your eyes, and breathe. Look to the right and look to the left three times, close your eyes, and breathe.

83. DIAGONAL RIGHT-LEFT
Look up diagonally to the right and diagonally down to the left three times, close your eyes, and breathe. Look up diagonally to the left and diagonally down to the right three times, close your eyes, and breathe.

84. AROUND THE CLOCK
Slowly look around the clock three times starting at twelve o'clock, then around to three, down to six, around to nine, and back up to twelve. Close your eyes and breathe. Slowly look around the clock counter clockwise three times starting at twelve o'clock, then around to nine, down to six, around to three, and then back up to twelve. Close your eyes and breathe.

85. FINGER GAZE
Starting with your index finger on the tip of your nose, slowly extend your arm and then return it to the start position, continually following your finger with your eyes. Lower your arm. Repeat three times. Close your eyes and breathe.

86. COVERED EYES
Remove glasses if needed. Rub the palms of your hands together, creating a little warmth. Close your eyes and place your hands on your cheekbones, covering but not touching your eyelids. Hold for three slow breaths. Lower your arms and relax the body.

FINAL RELAXATION AND MEDITATION

> *Watch your thoughts; they become words. Watch your words; they become actions. Watch your actions; they become habits. Watch your habits; they become character. Watch your character; for it becomes your destiny.*
>
> —Upanishads

Most yoga sessions finish with a period of relaxation. This can lead one to a meditative, sleepy, or unchanged state depending on any number of factors. It is best to keep in mind that relaxation does not need to be perfect, mind altering, or dramatic. The initial purpose of relaxation is to refresh the mind and absorb the benefits of your practice, just as you collect and regain your strength when you sleep. As you develop your practice, you may find that relaxation becomes many things to you, sometimes even something spiritual. If possible, let go of your initial expectations of what relaxation or meditation should be. Most importantly, give yourself permission to unwind and relax. Your final relaxation can be thought of as dessert. Rather than allowing your thoughts to drift toward things you will do after practice, savor each final moment as you would a delicious treat.

PREPARING TO RELAX
Allow your body to become still and relaxed, with your back pressing gently into the back of the chair. Rest your hands on your thighs in a comfortable position.

RELAXING BODY AND MIND
Complete relaxation takes practice and determination. By actively tensing then releasing muscles, it becomes easier to achieve.

FINAL RELAXATION AND MEDITATION

Squeeze your toes together, spread your toes apart, raise your feet an inch off the floor, and relax your feet. Squeeze your fingers together, spread your fingers apart, raise your arms an inch off your lap, and relax your arms. Squeeze your buttocks together, and then relax your buttocks. Squeeze your shoulders up to your ears, and then relax your shoulders. Open your mouth, stick your tongue out to your chin, and relax your face. Squeeze your face together, eyes, nose, and mouth, and then relax your face.

By the power of autosuggestion, relax your whole body:

I relax my toes, feet, calves, thighs, and hips.
I relax my fingers, hands, forearms, upper arms, shoulders, and shoulder blades.
I relax my back, neck, and face.
I relax my scalp, scull, and brain.
I relax my heart, lungs, liver, kidneys, and intestines.
All my inner organs are relaxed.
My body is relaxed.

MEDITATION
Sitting quietly and relaxing for a while after class may lead to meditation.

Repeating a mantra at the beginning of meditation helps to clear the mind. Choose any word or phrase that is meaningful and pleasing to you. For example, "Om," or "aum," which can be pronounced [haa ohhhh ng], is a universal mantra and is thought to have special qualities. Many believe that it is the underlying hum of all things in the universe. Om is used at the beginning and ending of many yoga classes.

To practice Om, begin with an inhalation, then breathy [ha-ohhh] on an exhalation. Near the end of the exhalation, make a long [ng] sound, which resonates through the nasal passages and upward.

ॐ THE Om SYMBOL

MEDITATION I
With each inhale, absorb the benefits of your practice: renewed muscles, bones, and skin; relaxed face and calm mind; and an overall balance of the self. With each exhale, let go a little more and release stress. Now allow any intentions or deliberate thoughts to melt away. Feel peace throughout the body and mind.

MEDITATION II
Visualize a large hourglass with the bottom full of small grains of sand. Turning the hourglass over in your mind, allow the sand to fall through the narrow midsection. Imagine that each grain of sand represents a perfect moment in your lifetime. Think how many thousands of perfect moments you have experienced and how very precious they are. Take a few moments to enjoy the warm feelings those memories bring.

Ending Your Relaxation/Meditation Phase:
Deepen your breath, start to wiggle your fingers and toes, and move your head from side to side. Take the arms up and overhead as you inhale. As you exhale, bring palms together at the heart.

Yoga classes sometimes end with a chant, such as Om, or a prayer. If desired, apply your own religious or spiritual prayers to your practice, or try this example from the Unity Church:

The Prayer for Protection
The light of God surrounds us; the love of God enfolds us;
The power of God protects us; the presence of God watches over us.
Wherever we are God is, and all is well.

NAMASTE

Namaste is a yoga greeting. It is usually said as one joins the palms together at the heart center and bows the head. This Sanskrit word translates to "I bow to you" and conveys "I see the divine spirit in you" or "I see a loving spirit in you." It is extended as an expression of respect.

> *There's only one corner of the universe you can be sure of changing, and that's your own self.*
> —Aldous Huxley

APPENDIX

SAMPLE SESSIONS

We describe a primary focus for each sequence, but your entire body will benefit from each practice. Begin each class with relaxation and a breathing exercise. End each class with a period of relaxation.

Session 1: All Seated
Use this sequence to develop a healthier posture, to strengthen upper-body muscles, and to enjoy a more open-heart center.

Pose Number	Pose Name
7	SHOULDER RELEASE
8	SIDE-TO-SIDE NECK WARM-UP
5	SHOULDER SHRUGS
6	SHOULDER ROLLS
4	CIRCLING ARMS
14	KNEE TO CHEST
64	ROCK THE BABY
65	PIGEON
1	CAT/COW
36	MOUNTAIN POSE
23	TRIANGLE
26	REVOLVED TRIANGLE
35	SPINAL TWIST
20	SUN SALUTATION
62	BACK OF SHOULDER STRETCH
63	MIDDLE OF BACK STETCH

APPENDIX

Session 2: All Seated
Use this sequence to strengthen your legs and core muscles.

Pose Number	Pose Name
18	FOOT ROTATIONS
15	LEG EXTENSIONS
12	KNEE LIFTS
3	FLOWING SPINAL TWIST
27	WARRIOR I
28	WARRIOR II
29	REVERSED WARRIOR
30	SIDE-ANGLE WARRIOR
33	EAGLE
23	TRIANGLE
26	REVOLVED TRIANGLE
64	ROCK THE BABY
65	PIGEON
66	HAMSTRING STRETCH
67	INNER THIGH STRETCH
2	FLOWING AIRPLANE

APPENDIX

Session 3: Seated and Standing
Use this sequence to improve balance and coordination.

Pose Number	Pose Name
17	TOE AND HEEL TAPPING
34	CHEST EXPANSION
35	SPINAL TWIST
51	BALANCE ON TOES
53	KNEE LIFTS
56	TREE
59	WARRIOR III
57	DANCER'S POSE
58	DANCER WITH HALF BOW
41	TRIANGLE
42	REVOLVED TRIANGLE
31	CAMEL
48	DOWNDOG
11	HALF MOON
68	WRIST RELEASE
70	LION POSE
69	FACIAL RELEASE

APPENDIX

Session 4: Seated and Standing
Acquire deeper flexibility and balance through the following sequence.

Pose Number	Pose Name
10	NECK PENDULUM
14	KNEE TO CHEST
21	CHAIR POSE
22	ARM CIRCLES
37	CAT/COW
39	PRAYER SQUAT FLOW
60	CHAIR SQUAT
61	CHAIR SQUAT ON ONE LEG
56	TREE
59	WARRIOR III
57	DANCER'S POSE
58	DANCER WITH HALF BOW
49	LEG RAISE
32	GATE
33	EAGLE
17	TOE AND HEEL TAPPING
18	FOOT ROTATIONS

APPENDIX

Session 5: Mostly Standing

Use this sequence to improve energy levels, increase back and chest flexibility, and to open the hips.

Pose Number	Pose Name
4	CIRCLING ARMS
17	TOE AND HEEL TAPPING
33	EAGLE
39	PRAYER SQUAT FLOW
49	LEG RAISE
41	TRIANGLE
42	REVOLVED TRIANGLE
51	BALANCE ON TOES
53	KNEE LIFTS
55	KNEE UP TWIST
54	KNEE TO CHEST
56	TREE
59	WARRIOR III
48	DOWNDOG
37	CAT/COW
52	FLAMINGO
50	FORWARD BEND
67	INNER THIGH STRETCH
64	ROCK THE BABY
65	PIGEON
71	SEATED FORWARD BEND

APPENDIX

Session 6: Mostly Standing

This sequence has the potential to build up heat, burn calories, and challenge your balance.

Pose Number	Pose Name
1	CAT/COW
16	ANKLE ROTATIONS
3	FLOWING SPINAL TWIST
36	MOUNTAIN POSE
43	WARRIOR I
44	WARRIOR II
45	REVERSED WARRIOR
46	SIDE-ANGLE WARRIOR
56	TREE
57	DANCER'S POSE
58	DANCER WITH HALF BOW
54	KNEE TO CHEST
60	CHAIR SQUAT
61	CHAIR SQUAT ON ONE LEG
37	CAT/COW
38	ARM CIRCLES
40	HALF MOON
47	CAMEL
13	KNEE CROSS AND ROTATE
72	FINGER FLEX
67	INNER THIGH STRETCH

APPENDIX

SANSKRIT NAMES

Alternate Nostril Breathing	*Anuloma Viloma*
Breathing Exercises	*Pranayama*
Camel	*Ustrasana*
Cat Pose	*Marjaryasana*
Chair Squat	*Utkatasana*
Cow	*Bitilasana*
Dancer's Pose	*Natarajasana*
Downdog	*Adho Mukha Svanasana*
Eagle	*Garudasana*
Easy Pose	*Sukhasana*
Extended Side-Angle Pose	*Utthita Parsvakonasana*
Gate Pose	*Parighasana*
Half Moon	*Ardha Chandrasana*
Lion Pose	*Simhasana*
Mountain Pose	*Tadasana*
Pigeon	*Eka Pada Rajakapotasana*
Posture	*Asana*
Revolved Triangle	*Parivrtta Trikonasana*
Seated Forward Bend	*Paschimottanasana*
Spinal Twist	*Ardha Matsyendrasana*
Standing Forward Bend	*Uttanasana*
Sun Salutation	*Surya Namaskar*
Tree	*Vrksasana*
Triangle	*Trikonasana*
Warrior	*Virabhadrasana*

RESOURCES

Bell, Lorna and Wudora Seyfer. Gentle Yoga. Cedar Rapids: Ingram Press, 1982.
   Gentle Yoga helps people with arthritis, stroke damage, multiple sclerosis, in wheelchairs, or anyone who needs a guide to yoga.

Christensen, Alice. The American Yoga Association Easy Does it Yoga. New York: Simon & Schuster, 1999.
   This is a complete yoga program for those challenged by age, illness, injury, or inactivity.

Dworkis, Sam. Recovery Yoga. New York: Three Rivers Press, 1997.
   Recovery Yoga addresses yoga for chronically ill, injured, and post-operative people.

Fishman, Loren and Ellen Saltonstall. Yoga for Arthritis. New York: W.W. Norton & Company, 2008.
   This is a collection of techniques that ease joint pain with yoga poses.

Kempton, Sally. "Letter to a New Meditator." Yoga Journal. September 2010: 77+

McGonigal, Kelly. "Your Brain on Meditation." Yoga Journal. June 2010: 69+
   These articles are helpful to anyone wanting a guide for practicing meditation.

Sweeney, Matthew. Ashtanga Yoga as It Is. The Yoga Temple, 2005.
   Sweeney outlines detailed information and photos showing the primary, intermediate, advanced A and B asanas, and vinyasa.

Vishnu-devananda, Swami. The Complete Illustrated Book of Yoga. New York: Crown Publisher, 1988.
   This book describes the benefits of yoga for the body, mind, and spirit.

© Clarissa C. Adkins, Olivette Baugh Robinson & Barbara Leaf Stewart 2010

Made in the USA
San Bernardino, CA
27 February 2014